FERTILITY DIET RECIPES FOR WOMEN

4 ULTIMATE DIET AND LIFESTYLE HACKS TO IMPROVE YOUR FERTILITY

Dr. Robin Howell

Table of contents

INTRODUCTION

UNDERSTANDING FERTILITY AND THE ROLE OF DIET

Fertility refers to a person's ability to conceive and have children. Fertility can be affected by a variety of factors, including age, medical conditions, lifestyle habits, and diet.

For women, fertility begins to decline in the late 20s and early 30s, and it continues to decrease as a woman gets older. This is due in part to the fact that a woman is born with all the eggs she will ever have, and the number and quality of those eggs decreases over time.

For men, fertility can also decline with age, although it tends to happen more gradually than it does in women. Medical conditions, such as testicular or prostate cancer, and certain lifestyle habits, such as smoking, can also affect male fertility.

If you are trying to get pregnant and are having difficulty, there are several things you can try to improve your fertility, such as maintaining a healthy diet and weight, managing stress, getting regular exercise, and avoiding tobacco and alcohol. If you have been trying to get pregnant for a year or more without success, or if you are over the age of 35 and have been trying for six months or more, it may be a good idea to speak with a healthcare provider for further evaluation and guidance

There are several factors that can affect fertility, and diet is just one of them. However, maintaining a healthy diet can be an important part of supporting fertility for both men and women.

For women, having a healthy weight is important for fertility. Being overweight or obese can lead to irregular periods and make it more difficult to get pregnant. On the other hand, being underweight can also disrupt menstrual cycles and reduce fertility. A balanced diet that includes a variety of nutrient-dense foods, such as fruits, vegetables, whole grains, and lean proteins, can help support a healthy weight and fertility.

For men, a healthy diet can also play a role in fertility. Some research suggests that a diet high in processed meats and full-fat dairy products may be associated with a lower sperm count and reduced fertility. On the other hand, a diet that includes a variety of fruits and vegetables, as well as healthy fats like those found in nuts and avocados, may support healthy sperm production.

It's also important to note that fertility can be affected by other factors, such as age, medical conditions, and lifestyle factors like

stress and alcohol consumption. If you have concerns about your fertility, it's a good idea to speak with a healthcare provider for personalized advice..

Diet can play a role in fertility for both men and women. Here are a few ways that diet can affect fertility:

- Weight: For women, being at a healthy weight can increase fertility. Being overweight or obese can disrupt menstrual cycles and make it more difficult to get pregnant. On the other hand, being underweight can also cause irregular periods and reduce fertility. A balanced diet that includes a variety of nutrient-dense foods, such as fruits, vegetables, whole grains, and lean proteins, can help support a healthy weight and fertility.
- Nutrient deficiencies: Certain nutrient deficiencies, such as low levels of iron, folic acid, and vitamin D, can affect fertility. A diet that includes a variety of nutrient-rich foods can help ensure that you are getting all the nutrients you need to support fertility.
- Processed foods and unhealthy fats: A diet high in processed foods and unhealthy fats, such as trans fats and saturated fats, may be associated with a lower sperm count and reduced fertility in men.
- Antioxidants: Some research suggests that a diet rich in antioxidants, such as those found in fruits and vegetables, may improve fertility by reducing oxidative stress in the body.

It's important to note that diet is just one factor that can affect fertility, and it's not always possible to improve fertility through diet alone. If you have concerns about your fertility, it's a good idea to speak with a healthcare provider for personalized advice..

BENEFITS OF FOLLOWING A FERTILITY DIET

There is some evidence to suggest that following a fertility diet may improve reproductive health and increase the likelihood of pregnancy. Some potential benefits include:

- Maintaining a healthy weight: Being overweight or obese can affect fertility in both men and women. A fertility diet may help you maintain a healthy weight, which can improve your chances of conceiving.

- Getting enough nutrients: A fertility diet can help you get the nutrients you need, such as folic acid, iron, and calcium, which are important for reproductive health.
- Reducing inflammation: Inflammation can affect fertility, and some foods can contribute to inflammation in the body. A fertility diet may help reduce inflammation by including anti-inflammatory foods, such as fatty fish, nuts, and leafy greens.
- Improving insulin sensitivity: Insulin resistance can affect fertility, and a diet that helps improve insulin sensitivity may improve your chances of conceiving.
- Reducing the risk of certain health conditions: Some health conditions, such as polycystic ovary syndrome (PCOS) and endometriosis, can affect fertility. A fertility diet may help reduce the risk of these conditions by including certain nutrients and limiting others.
- Limiting alcohol intake: Excessive alcohol consumption can affect fertility in both men and women. A fertility diet may recommend limiting alcohol intake or avoiding it altogether to improve reproductive health.
- Reducing caffeine intake: While it's not clear if caffeine directly affects fertility, some studies have suggested that high caffeine intake may slightly reduce the chances of getting pregnant. A fertility diet may recommend limiting caffeine intake to 200 mg or less per day.
- Incorporating fertility-boosting foods: Some foods, such as leafy greens, berries, and nuts, may have fertility-boosting properties due to their nutrient content. A fertility diet may include these types of foods to potentially improve reproductive health

It's important to note that while a fertility diet may have potential benefits, it's not a guarantee of pregnancy and should be used in combination with other fertility treatments as recommended by a healthcare provider.

HOW TO USE THIS BOOK

Congratulations, you got the right book at the right time for your fertility diet cookbook and plans, here are a few general tips for using this book:

- Follow the plan as directed: It's important to follow the plan as closely as possible to get the full benefits of the fertility diet. This may include following specific meal plans, recipes, and guidelines for food and nutrient intake.
- Consult with a healthcare provider: Before starting any new diet, it's always a good idea to consult with a healthcare provider, especially if you have any existing health conditions or are pregnant or trying to become pregnant. Your healthcare provider can help you determine if the fertility diet is safe and appropriate for you.
- Make adjustments as needed: It's okay to make adjustments to the fertility diet if you find certain recipes or meal plans don't work for you. Just be sure to keep the overall principles of the diet in mind and try to find substitutes that align with the plan.
- Don't rely on the fertility diet alone: While a fertility diet may have potential benefits, it's not a guarantee of pregnancy and should be used in combination with other fertility treatments as recommended by a healthcare provider.
- Enjoy the process: Cooking and eating can be a fun and enjoyable experience, so try to make the most of it! Experiment with new recipes and ingredients, and don't be afraid to get creative in the kitchen

CHAPTER ONE

FERTILITY-BOOSTING NUTRIENTS

1. Folic acid

Folic acid is a B vitamin that is essential for proper brain function and plays a key role in mental and emotional health. It is also important for the production of red blood cells and the metabolism of homocysteine. Adequate intake of folic acid is particularly important during periods of rapid growth, such as infancy, adolescence, and pregnancy. It can be found in a variety of foods, including leafy green vegetables, citrus fruits, beans, and grains.

Folic acid is a type of B vitamin that is important for proper brain function and plays a key role in mental and emotional health. It is also important for women who are trying to get pregnant because it can help to prevent birth defects in the baby's brain and spine. Taking folic acid before and during pregnancy can also help to reduce the risk of preterm labor and low birth weight. Some studies have also suggested that folic acid may help to improve fertility by reducing the risk of ovulatory failure and improving the quality of the eggs. It is important to talk to a healthcare provider about the

recommended dosage of folic acid and the best way to incorporate it into your diet.

Certainly! Here are a few more things you might want to know about folic acid and fertility:

- The recommended daily intake of folic acid for women who are planning to become pregnant is 400 micrograms (mcg). This can be obtained through a combination of diet and supplements. Good dietary sources of folic acid include leafy green vegetables, citrus fruits, beans, and whole grains.
- Folic acid is especially important in the first few weeks of pregnancy, when the neural tube is forming. This is why it is important for women to start taking folic acid before they become pregnant. If a woman does not get enough folic acid before and during pregnancy, it can increase the risk of birth defects known as neural tube defects.
- Some studies have suggested that taking folic acid may also help to improve fertility in women with certain conditions, such as polycystic ovary syndrome (PCOS) or endometriosis.

- It is important to talk to a healthcare provider before taking any supplements, including folic acid. This is especially important if you are taking any medications, as some medications can interact with supplements. A healthcare provider can help you
determine the right dosage and advise you on any potential risks or interactions.
- Folic acid is not the only nutrient that is important for fertility. A healthy diet that is rich in a variety of nutrients, including vitamins, minerals, and antioxidants, can help to support fertility. Some other nutrients that are important for fertility include iron, zinc, and omega-3 fatty acids.
- Maintaining a healthy weight is also important for fertility. Being overweight or underweight can affect hormone levels and ovulation, which can make it more difficult to get pregnant.
- Managing stress can also be important for fertility. High levels of stress can interfere with hormone levels and disrupt ovulation. It can be helpful to find ways to manage stress, such as through exercise, relaxation techniques, or therapy.

If you are having difficulty getting pregnant, it is important to talk to a healthcare provider. They can help you to understand the potential causes of fertility issues and recommend treatment options, if necessary

2. Iron

Iron is an essential nutrient that is necessary for the production of red blood cells, which carry oxygen throughout the body. It is also
needed for the synthesis of collagen, a protein that helps to form connective tissue, and for the proper functioning of the immune system. Iron is found in a variety of foods, including red meat, poultry, seafood, beans, lentils, nuts, seeds, and leafy green vegetables. The recommended daily intake of iron for adult men and women is 8 mg and 18 mg, respectively. However, people who are pregnant or have certain medical conditions may need more. It is important to consume enough iron to prevent anemia, which is a condition characterized by a deficiency of red blood cells or hemoglobin, the protein in red blood cells that carries

oxygen. If you think you may be low in iron, it is a good idea to talk to your doctor or a registered dietitian.

There are two forms of dietary iron: heme and non-heme. Heme iron is found in animal sources, such as red meat, poultry, and seafood, and is more easily absorbed by the body. Non-heme iron is found in plant-based sources, such as beans, lentils, nuts, seeds, and leafy green vegetables, and is not as well absorbed. Vitamin C can help to increase the absorption of nonheme iron. So, eating iron-rich foods along with foods that are high in vitamin C, like citrus fruits, can be helpful. Calcium can interfere with the absorption of iron. So, it's a good idea to avoid consuming large amounts of calcium-rich foods (such as dairy products) at the same time as iron-rich foods. Some medications, such as antacids and some types of pain relievers, can interfere with the absorption of iron. If you are taking any medications, it is important to talk to your doctor or pharmacist about any potential interactions with iron. If you are concerned about your iron intake or are at risk for anemia, it is a good idea to talk to your doctor or a registered dietitian. They can help you to determine if you need to take an iron supplement and can provide guidance on how to get enough iron from your diet.

In women, iron is necessary for the production of estrogen, a hormone that plays a role in the menstrual cycle and fertility. A deficiency in iron can disrupt the menstrual cycle and lead to anemia, which can affect fertility. Adequate iron intake may also be important for the development of a healthy pregnancy.

In men, iron is necessary for the production of sperm. A deficiency in iron may lead to a decrease in sperm count and fertility.

It is important for both men and women to consume enough iron to support fertility and overall health. If you are concerned about your iron intake or fertility, it is a good idea to talk to your doctor or a registered dietitian. They can help you to determine if you need to take an iron supplement and can provide guidance on how to get enough iron from your diet.

3. Zinc

Zinc is an essential nutrient that is necessary for the proper functioning of the immune system, wound healing, taste and smell, and DNA synthesis. It is also involved in the metabolism of carbohydrates, proteins, and fats. Zinc is found in a wide variety of foods, including red meat, poultry, seafood, beans, nuts, and whole grains. It is also available as a dietary supplement.

Some people may be at risk of zinc deficiency, including vegetarians and vegans, people with digestive disorders, and those with malabsorption conditions. Zinc deficiency can lead to a number of health problems, including impaired growth and development, diarrhea, and impaired immune function.

If you are concerned about your zinc intake, you should speak to a healthcare professional. They can assess your dietary intake and determine if you need a supplement. It is important to follow the recommended daily intake for zinc and not exceed the upper limit, as excessive zinc can interfere with the absorption of other minerals and may cause negative side effects.

4. Omega-3 fatty acids

Omega-3 fatty acids are a type of polyunsaturated fat that are essential for human health. They are called "essential" because the body cannot produce them on its own and must get them from the diet. Omega-3 fatty acids are important for maintaining heart health and have also been shown to have anti-inflammatory effects and to be beneficial for brain health. Some common sources of omega-3 fatty acids include fatty fish, such as salmon and mackerel, nuts and seeds, and vegetable oils. It is generally recommended that people

consume at least two servings of fatty fish per week to get enough omega-3 fatty acids.

There is some evidence to suggest that omega-3 fatty acids may be beneficial for fertility. For example, a review of studies found that higher intake of omega-3 fatty acids was associated with a higher likelihood of becoming pregnant and having a live birth in women undergoing assisted reproduction techniques, such as in vitro fertilization. Omega-3 fatty acids may also be beneficial for male fertility, as they have been shown to improve sperm quality and motility. However, it is important to note that more research is needed to fully understand the relationship between omega-3 fatty acids and fertility. As with any health issue, it is always best to consult with a healthcare provider for advice on how to optimize fertility.

There are several ways that omega-3 fatty acids may potentially be beneficial for fertility. Some research suggests that they may help to regulate menstrual cycles and improve the thickness of the uterine lining, both of which may be important for successful pregnancy. Omega-3 fatty acids may also have anti-inflammatory effects, and inflammation has been linked to fertility problems in both men and women. In addition, omega-3 fatty acids may have a positive effect on hormone balance, which is important for reproductive health.

It's worth noting that the relationship between omega-3 fatty acids and fertility is not fully understood, and more research is needed to determine the extent to which these fats may be beneficial.

CHAPTER TWO

MEAL PLANNING AND RECIPE IDEAS

Breakfast

1. **Fertility-Boosting Smoothie**

If you are trying to get pregnant and you aren't drinking a fertility smoothie everyday you are missing out! First, smoothies are delicious. Second, it's easy to pack them full of healthy greens, proteins, and fats, which are all very important to a healthy fertility diet. Finally, if you are struggling with specific types of infertility diagnosis, you can incorporate your healing superfood fertility "boosters" in your smoothies!

THE RULES OF FERTILITY SMOOTHIES

- RULE 1: EAT YOUR FLORA

Your diurnal fertility smoothie is the perfect way to make sure you get a redundant serving or two of the lush flora you need to boost your fertility! The salutary leafy flora include veggies similar to romaine, kale, spinach, collards, watercress, arugula, cabbage, beet flora, chards, and dandelion flora. These flora fight infertility by

creating a healthy sperm-friendly alkaline terrain and by furnishing pivotal minerals, antioxidants and vitamins that are demanded to grow healthy eggs and sustain a successful gestation. I recommend 2- 4 servings of flora a day(although one serving is from the nettles in your diurnal fertility herbal infusion), and it's much easier to get at least one of these servings in a smoothie.

One serving is equal to 1 mug raw, or ½ mug cooked dark green leafy vegetables.

Can I break this rule? Yes, but make sure you're eating a large green lettuce salad every day and two fresh cooked green veggies.

- RULE 2: AVOID- THESE-RAW- VEGGIES

There's the thing- for the utmost of the healthy leafy flora, you SHOULD NOT EAT THEM RAW. This includes in your smoothie. That's right- no more raw kale or spinach in your smoothies or in your salads. I know, I know, you suppose I 'm crazy. The other fertility websites say its okay. Well, they're wrong. the utmost of these raw leafy flora are veritably delicate to digest and you do n't want your body to use up its energy on digestion. You need your body to concentrate on making healthy eggs and circulating blood to the uterus. also, while Chinese Medicine(i.e., your acupuncturist) occasionally approves of a many raw veggies in the summer, for numerous infertility - related conditions similar as Cold Uterus, order Yang Deficiency, or any Damp conditions, no raw veggies are recommended.

So what are you to do? You need to smoothly foam any cruciferous vegetables which are veritably delicate on digestion arugula, cauliflower, cabbage, turnip, collard flora, bok choy, brussels sprouts, radishes, rutabaga, and watercress. You also need to smoothly foam any green veggies that are high in gut- prickly oxalic acid. These include spinach, chard, parsley, chives, purslane, and beet flora. Flora you can put in your smoothie raw include Romaine, Red or Green splint lettuce, or adulation lettuce.

Can I break this rule? Yes, plenitude of people get pregnant while blending raw spinach into their smoothies. It simply is n't optimal. I had a case with 5 different infertility opinion that she crushed by doing ALL THE effects and always optimizing my choices, so i employ you to follow this rule closely.However, do n't sweat this one, If you're just starting to try to conceive. This rule is the most important for women who have digestive issues of any kind, or have been diagnosed by their Traditional Chinese Medicine guru(acupuncturist) with Spleen Qi insufficiency, order Yang Deficiency, or Cold Uterus.

- RULE 3: ROTATE YOUR FLORA

Rotate your flora, people! Do n't put kale in your smoothie every day for a time. Not only is it not intriguing, but you're limiting your nutrients and minerals. It's also possible- although largely doubtful to have " alkaloid buildup " which can harm our thyroid. You can
indeed develop hypothyroidism from carousing on cruciferous veggies, like kale. When you smoothly foam your veggies, still, the goitens that produce the glucosinolates that affect the thyroid are incompletely destroyed by heat. So, brume down, and mix it up! Enjoy mixing it up by interspersing with raw lettuces, especially in the summer!

Can I break this rule? Yes, but you really should n't. It is n't healthy for your body to have the same food over and over every day!
What to do in your smoothies In the summer, rotate through raw organic romaine, green splint, or butterhead lettuces. For the other three seasons

buy frozen organic kale or spinach in bulk and smoothly foam a bunch for the week also store in a glass pyrex in the fridge to use in my smoothies. We use this high grade pristine sword vegetable steamer inside our non-toxic each- sheatheTri-Ply cookware. sometimes rotate these out for raw romaine, or smoothly fumed collards, watercress, or chard.

- RULE 4: WATCH YOUR SUGARS

It's too easy to go crazy with fruit when you make your smoothies, not to mention how numerous people add fresh sweeteners similar to honey to their smoothies. To maximize egg health you need to keep your insulin response on an even ship. So if you're putting a banana, mango, and some pineapple in your smoothie, you're
putting your body into sugar shock which can affect your egg health.

Sugars are also sneaky and can show up in other ways, like as a component in your protein greasepaint that you did n't indeed realize was there. Then's the thing- all sugar is problematic for fertility and egg health, indeed when it comes as natural fructose in fruit. This means that you ca n't trust constituents that would typically be okay in a " clean " eating diet similar as honey, agave, or maple saccharinity.
What should you do? Choose fruits with low overall sugar(not just low- glycemic fruit) and a high- antioxidant or fiber content, similar to apples, pears, and berries. Limit your total fruit consumption to 2- 3 servings a day, or 1- 2 if you have PCOS and need to control your blood sugar situations more closely. 1 serving = 1 medium fruit(baseball sized) or ½ mug diced fruit.

Can I break this rule? If you're under 35, have been trying to conceive for a time, have no enterprises about egg quality, and don't have Polycystic Ovarian Pattern(PCOS), also yes, you can break this rule. Heck, if you're 26 and just started trying, feel free to load your smoothie up with bananas, mangoes, and perhaps indeed throw in a little organic blackstrap molasses for fresh agreeableness and vitamins. Still, if you have PCOS, high FSH,

low AMH, a history of repeated early confinement or chemical infertility , or any other kind
of infertility struggle that might be related to egg quality, do n't break this rule.

 What to do in your smoothies rotate through organic berries: blueberries, snorts, strawberries, blackberries, and sometimes in half a small green apple if you are pining a little redundant agreeableness. To save plutocrats you can generally buy bulk frozen organic berries- indeed though fresh would be better it's truly prohibitive for a diurnal smoothie. This is the only frozen item in any of my smoothies.

 RULE 5: DO NOT GO FROZEN!

In Chinese Medicine, cold foods(including foods that are literally " cold ") can chill the uterus and make it an unpleasant place for an embryo to implant. Ladies, we want our uteruses to be warm jungles packed with love and nutrients for our little babies to- be. This means you need to avoid icy smoothies. Whenever possible, keep constituents at room temperature(fruit, veggies,etc.), and avoid frozen constituents.

 Can you break this rule? Yes, plenty of women get pregnant while drinking icy potables daily. It just is n't ideal, and by now you know me you can always shoot for optimizing all my fertility opinions. This rule is the most important for women with Traditional Chinese drug opinion of order Yang Deficiency, Spleen Qi Deficiency, Blood Stasis, or Cold Uterus.

MY FERTILITY SMOOTHIE FORM FOR HIGH FSH, ENDOMETRIOSIS, EGG QUALITY(LOW AMH, LOW ANTRAL FOLLICLE COUNT & REPEATED EARLY LOSS)

- 1 mug organic romaine or adulation lettuce, or1/2 mug smoothly fumed spinach or kale(collards or chard if you're stalwart)
- /2 mug- 1 mug organic berries(fresh preferable, frozen if you ca n't go fresh or they're out of season)

- 2 scoops Perfect Supplements Hydrolyzed Collagen
- Tbsp organic walnut oil painting(further if you're going Keto)(for my endometriosis- use another fat suited to YOUR requirements)
- 1 scoop wheatgrass greasepaint(for my High FSH and acupuncture judgments use a superfood suited to YOUR requirements)
- 1 tsp spirulina(for my poor egg quality and acupuncture judgments use a superfood suited to YOUR requirements)
- 1 Scoop Acai greasepaint
- mug thin SO Coconut Milk(or, enough to fill to the " Fill " line on your Nutribullet) OR filtered water OR indeed more your own manual coconut or nut milk

Instructions
Add all the constituents to your NutriBullet, or other blender, and mix for 30 seconds or so. Enjoy!

FERTILITY SMOOTHIE FOR EGG HEALTH

This is the fertility smoothie I gave to a case to drink every day to get pregnant despite endometriosis, High FSH, low AMH, lowered ovarian reserve, MTHFR single mutation, and repeated deliveries. The focus was on perfecting egg health overall, and prostrating my individual issues. Be sure to change out MY superfoods(e.g., walnut oil painting for endometriosis, wheatgrass for High FSH,etc.,) for YOUR particular situation!

- 1 mug organic romaine or adulation lettuce, or1/2 mug smoothly fumed spinach or kale(collards or chard if you 're stalwart)
- / 2 mug – 1 mug organic berries(fresh preferable, frozen if you ca n't go fresh or they're out of season)
- scoops Perfect Supplements Hydrolyzed Collagen
- 1 scoop wheatgrass greasepaint(for my High and acupuncture judgments use a superfood suited to YOUR requirements)
- 1 tsp spirulina(for my poor egg quality and acupuncture judgments use a superfood suited to YOUR requirements)

- mug filtered water(or whatever you need to reach the filler line on your Nutribullet)
- 2 tbsp coconut manna
- 1 scoop acai greasepaint

INSTRUCTIONS

Add all constituents to your NutriBullet, or other blender, and mix for 30 seconds or so.

Enjoy!

NOTES

You can sub whatever kind of thin coconut/ almond milk,etc., for the water coconut manna quintet. I 'm just trying to avoid using mimetic or tetra pak milks with epoxies in them, so I 'm making my own coconut milk with the manna in a glass jar plus water.

Occasionally you can add half an apple.

First try removing the wheatgrass and spirulina, If this is too not- tasty for you. Is it good also? If it still is n't tasty, switch to romaine rather of smoothly fumed spinach or kale. Is it good also? Introduce other particulars until its tasty enough! You WILL get used to it, I promise! DO N'T ADD THE BANANA.

Have fun! Play around with different combinations. Throw some seeds or nuts in if you want. Just watch your sugars, i.e., do n't throw in the banana!

SEED CYCLING IN YOUR FERTILITY SMOOTHIE

Still, the easiest way to get the ground seeds into your diet is by adding them to your smoothie! You can check out my whole post on
Seed Cycling for Fertility then, If you're looking into seed cycling for balancing your hormones or boosting fertility.

That's my general seed cycling protocol

CD1- CD14 OR OVULATION(MENSTRUAL & FOLLICULAR PHASE)

- 1 Tbsp organic flax seeds, lately base in my smoothie
- Tbsp organic pumpkin seeds(peeled), lately base in my smoothie

CD15 OR OVULATION- END OF CYCLE,I.E., MY PERIOD CAME(LUTEAL PHASE)

- 1 Tbsp organic sesame seeds, lately base in my smoothie
- 1 Tbsp organic sunflower seeds, lately base in my smoothie

NOTES ON THE FERTILITY SMOOTHIE

Now that you 've made it through my total post on fertility smoothies, I hope YOU are not exhausted! My form is below, please enjoy, and make it YOURS. Just like the Fertility Diet, the Fertility Smoothie should be acclimatized to your particular situation(and tastes!).

A quick note on taste — ladies, this smoothie isn't going to taste like the bones you 've made with two bananas, mangoes, honey, and whole fat dairy.
Note- you can make your smoothie a little bit each day. occasionally you can have a raw gusto/ blueberries/ lime juice quintet. occasionally you can also add snorts, a little bit of gojis, and add some cocoa greasepaint. It all depends on the day and what I 'm feeling. This is the introductory smoothie that I recommend for my cases with High FSH, endometriosis, Low AMH, lowered ovarian reserve, and MTHFR mutation. It was one of the 79 effects I recommend to get pregnant!

2. EGG AND VEGETABLE BREAKFAST SCRAMBLE

Healthy Veggie Egg Scramble is a succulent breakfast or easy regale filled with veggies and ready in no time, then it is! The stylish egg scramble loaded with healthy veggies! A great way to use up your veggies in the fridge to make stylish climbed eggs and veggies! Ready in lower than 30 twinkles!

Then's a form for an egg and vegetable breakfast scramble
Ingredients

- 2 eggs
- 1/2 mug minced vegetables(similar as bell peppers, onions, and mushrooms)
- tbsp adulation or oil painting
- swab and pepper to taste

Instructions

- toast a small visage over medium heat and add the adulation or oil painting.
- When the adulation is melted or the oil painting is hot, add the minced vegetables to the visage and cook until they're tender, about 5 twinkles.
- Beat the eggs in a small coliseum and season with swab and pepper.
- Pour the eggs over the vegetables in the visage and scramble until the eggs are cooked to your asked doneness.
- Serve the scramble incontinently, garnished with fresh swab and pepper if asked .

This scramble is a quick and easy breakfast option that can be customized with your favorite vegetables. You can also add rubbish, sauces, or minced cooked meat to the scramble if you like. Enjoy!

Ingredients
- Tbsp adulation
- bell pepper, minced
- mugs spinach
- 2 large eggs
- 6 grape tomatoes, sliced in half
- 1/ 4 avocado, sliced
- 1/ 4 mug hummus
- pinch Swab and pepper

INSTRUCTIONS

Add the adulation to a large non-stick skillet and heat over medium. Once melted, add the minced bell pepper and sauté for 1- 2 twinkles. Add the spinach and sauté just until wilted(about one nanosecond).

Push the vegetable to the sides and crack the eggs in the center. Add the seasoning of your choice. Keeping the skillet over medium heat, begin to scramble the eggs, mixing them with the vegetables. When the eggs are substantially set, remove the skillet from the heat.

Add the cooked eggs and vegetables to a coliseum and top with sliced tomatoes, avocado, hummus, and a pinch of swab and pepper. Serve incontinently.

8 VEGETABLES THAT GO WITH EGGS

Start your day on a positive note with a savory, nutritional breakfast of eggs and veggies. Or, enjoy this creation at any time of day.However, browse this succulent list for a plenitude of ideas!

If you're wondering what vegetables pair well with eggs and dishes you can make.

1. SPINACH

There are numerous ways to incorporate spinach into your egg dishes, from mixing spinach into your climbed eggs to making a succulent leafy green frittata. Spinach adds a rich cure of vitamins like A, C, K, iron, and potassium, making it a nutritional and scrumptious addition to your mess.

still, then are a many ideas to get you started

If you 're looking for ways to combine eggs and spinach. climbed eggs with spinach A quick and simple yet delicious mess, climbed eggs with spinach is an excellent way to start the day with a nutritional breakfast. With savory spinach, climbed organic eggs, grated parmesan and mozzarella, and plenty of fresh spices, you'll enjoy your morning the right way with a healthy and succulent mess.

Spinach, black bean and egg quesadillas Whether you need a nutritional breakfast for the family or a quick weeknight regale to pull together, these

egg quesadillas with spinach and black sap are a great result. Try adding some hot sauce or a nugget of sour cream for a redundant burst of flavor.
 Spinach and rubbish strata You ca n't go wrong with a savory quintet of eggs, spinach, chuck and rubbish — that's why this spinach and rubbish strata is ideal for any time of the day. Try it out for your coming mess!
2. TOMATOES
 Sweet, juicy, and full of antioxidants, tomatoes are another great food to brace with eggs. Plus, there are endless ways to do so! Whether mixing fresh tomatoes and hard- boiled eggs in a salad, making a succulent sandwich, or using these two ingredients in a hearty haze, you can produce the ultimate savory mess with tomatoes and eggs. Below are some fashions to help you along

 Egg, lettuce, and tomato sandwich You 're presumably familiar with the classic BLT sandwich, but get ready to meet the ELT Supreme! This sandwich combines whole- grain or wheat chuck, crisp iceberg lettuce, fresh tomato, and egg for a wholly scrumptious meal.However, mess, and calories, If you want the succulent taste of a BLT minus the added fat.
 Easy classic omelet Breakfast is the most important mess of the day, and there's no better way to rise and shine than with a classic egg omelet. With numerous eggs, fresh cilantro and parsley, grated parmesan, minced onions and peppers and of course, tomatoes you can whip up this succulent dish in beats.
 Roasted ratatouille with eggs A traditional French dish that began in the 1800s, ratatouille is a savory comfort mess composed of
thinly sliced vegetables on a bed of tomato sauce. There are multitudinous variations of this dish, and this bone includes a unique twist — eggs. This roasted ratatouille with eggs combines fresh tomatoes, eggplant, zucchini, and other veggies and spices for a rich burst of flavor. Mealtime is sure to be a delight with this form!
 3. GREEN ONIONS
 An excellent source of sulfur and other essential nutrients, green onions brace wonderfully with egg dishes to boost their overall nutrition. Not to mention they 're vital for adding flavor and scent to various fashions.

Learn further about how you can combine green onions and eggs with the dishes below

Egg white and foliage frittata If you want a mess that cuts down on calories and cholesterol, an egg white and foliage frittata provides an optimal boost of nutrition and energy in the morning. This dish includes spinach, peppers, green onions, scallions, egg whites, and other fresh ingredients for a succulent green breakfast.

Southwestern egg rolls Enjoy the flavors of southwestern cookery and the perfect crunch of egg rolls with this succulent dish. These southwestern egg rolls combine climbed eggs, minced green onions, tattered Monterey jack rubbish, and other fresh veggies and spices all packed into a crisp fried tortilla shell.

Fresh Theater vegetable dish Whether you 're cooking for the family or bringing a dish to a potluck, this fresh theater vegetable dish is sure to be a megahit. snare cornucopia of eggs, two stalks of minced green onions, some Italian seasoning, and the other ingredients on the list and give this appetizing form a pass!

4. PEPPERS

Low in calories and an excellent source of fiber, vitamins A and C, and other nutrients, peppers are a precious addition to multitudinous reflections. Whether you prefer green, red or pusillanimous bell peppers or indeed salty jalapenos — there are various ways to add peppers to egg dishes. Browse the fashions below for some ideas

Jalapeno popper egg mugs No matter the occasion — whether a simple family mess, party, or potluck — these jalapeno popper egg mugs presumably wo n't last long. They 're fun to eat and give a nutritive mix of flavors. With minced jalapeno peppers, fresh eggs, cool sour cream, and other succulent ingredients, youths and grown- ups likewise are sure to enjoy these savory culinary delights.

rubbish, bacon and egg millions Amp up breakfast time with these millions with bacon and rubbish. Green pepper, fresh eggs, sizzling bacon, tattered rubbish, and enchilada sauce will surely start your day on a high note.

Spinach and pepper fried egg flatbread Indulge in recently grilled eggs and vegetables sautéed to perfection when you stink into this spinach and pepper fried egg flatbread. This dish combines crisp vegetables, recently squeezed lemon juice, spices, eggs, and flatbread for warm, rich flavors. Start your morning right by combining classic ingredients and gravies into a uniquely succulent breakfast!

5. AVOCADO

Smooth, savory and full of flavor, avocados add the perfect touch of texture and taste to multitudinous dishes. They 're also rich in magnesium, potassium, vitamins B6, C, E, and more! Consider adding avocado to your egg dishes for an excellent source of nutrients and flavor.However, we 've listed some below

If you 're looking for egg and avocadofashions.Avocado toast This is a popular breakfast choice and for good reason. It's both succulent and easy to whip up in the mornings. All you need are a numerous ingredients — two ripe avocados, fresh eggs, chuck

, pepper, and minced chives. This simple avocado toast with soft- boiled egg is sure to become a favorite breakfast in your home!

Eggs baked in avocado This unique breakfast will surely spark your interest if you 're an addict of avocados and trying interesting fashions. These eggs burned in avocado combine eggs, bacon bits, recently base black pepper, and minced chives all burned into a fresh avocado.However, consider giving this dish a pass, If you have a little spare time in the morning to pop a mess into the rotisserie.

Climbed eggs, avocado, and smoked salmon climbed eggs are formerly succulent on their own — but Texas toast, protein-rich salmon, and delicate avocado make them indeed more! Try out these climbed eggs with avocado and smoked salmon for your coming mess.

6. SWEET POTATOES

Sweet potatoes are rich, tasteful, and a vitaminA-rich volition to regular potatoes. They add just the right mix of sweet and savory flavors to your plate, making them succulent for any mess of the day.However, check out the ideas we 've listed below

If you 're wondering how to add sweet potatoes to your egg dishes.

Sweet potato, savant, and egg tacos Ideal for both family feasts and breakfasts, these tacos with sweet potatoes and eggs are packed with protein and easy to whip up. With some warm tortillas, sweet potatoes, fresh savant, eggs, and tattered rubbish, you 'll have a succulent mess for everyone in under an hour.

Sweet potato Brussels sow skillet This form blends fresh sweet potato, Brussels sprouts, white onions, mushrooms, eggs, and fresh spices for an ultra-savory quintet. Start your day with this succulent sweet potato Brussels sprouts skillet!

Sweet potato hash with fried eggs If a sweet and rich yet savory breakfast sounds charming, consider trying out this sweet potato hash with fried eggs. Sweet potatoes, onion, baby spinach, and crisp bell pepper give way to fresh spices and sizzling fried eggs for inconceivable flavor.However, this mess is ideal, If you need a succulent morning pick- me- up before heading to work.

7. POTATOES

a phenomenal source of fiber and flavor, it's no surprise that potatoes are a favorite food for many. With this protean veggie, you can whip up numerous succulent fashions, from breakfast burritos to regale casseroles.However, then are some dishes to try out

If you need help deciding what to make with eggs and potatoes.

Summer salad with eggs Nothing says summer relatively like a cool, crisp, and refreshing salad. This is a healthy, energy- boosting quintet of romaine lettuce, arugula flora, and red, white, and blue baby potatoes. No matter the time of day, this summer salad with eggs form is a nutritional addition to your mess.

introductory fried eggs and potatoes protest off your day with a simple, classic, and wholly American breakfast. This introductory fried eggs and potatoes form is perfect if you 're looking for a delicious, easy- to- make mess in the morning. Chances are, you 'll formerly have the utmost of these constituents sitting in your kitchen!

Egg and rubbish stuffed ignited potatoes This dish is incredibly easy to make in bulk if you 're hosting brunch. snare some medium potatoes, thick- cut bacon, eggs, green onion, and cheddar rubbish to give this form a go! These egg and rubbish stuffed ignited potatoes are sure to impress potato suckers and indeed the pickiest of guests

LUNCH

1. **Fertility-Boosting Salad**

There are many potential ingredients that could be included in a fertility-boosting salad. Here are a few ideas:

- Leafy greens such as spinach, kale, and arugula, which are rich in folate and other nutrients that are important for fertility.
- Cruciferous vegetables like broccoli, cauliflower, and Brussels sprouts, which contain compounds that may help to regulate estrogen and other hormones.
- Citrus fruits like oranges, lemons, and grapefruits, which are high in vitamin C and may help to improve sperm quality.
- Avocado, which is a good source of healthy fats and nutrients like vitamin E, which is important for reproductive health.
- Nuts and seeds like almonds, pumpkin seeds, and flaxseeds, which are rich in omega-3 fatty acids and other nutrients that may help to support fertility.
- Legumes like beans, lentils, and chickpeas, which are high in protein and fiber and may help to regulate hormones.
- Whole grains like quinoa, brown rice, and oats, which are rich in B vitamins and other nutrients that are important for fertility.

Remember that everyone's nutritional needs are different, so it's important to speak with a healthcare provider or a registered dietitian to determine the best diet for your specific needs

There are many different ingredients that have been claimed to have fertility-boosting properties, so there are many different ways that you could make a fertility-boosting salad. Here is one recipe that you could try:

(1)

Ingredients:
- 1/2 cup quinoa
- 1 cup water
- 1 cup cherry tomatoes, halved
- 1/2 cup diced cucumber
- 1/2 cup diced red bell pepper
- 1/4 cup diced red onion
- 1/4 cup crumbled feta cheese
- 2 tablespoons chopped fresh parsley
- 2 tablespoons olive oil
- 1 tablespoon red wine vinegar
- Salt and pepper to taste

Directions:
- Rinse the quinoa in a fine mesh strainer and then add it to a small saucepan with the water. Bring to a boil, then reduce the heat to low and simmer, covered, until the quinoa is tender and the water has been absorbed, about 15-20 minutes.
- Allow the quinoa to cool to room temperature.
- In a large bowl, combine the cherry tomatoes, cucumber, red bell pepper, red onion, feta cheese, and parsley.
- Add the cooled quinoa to the bowl with the vegetables and toss to combine.
- In a small bowl, whisk together the olive oil, red wine vinegar, salt, and pepper.
- Pour the dressing over the salad and toss to coat.
- Serve the salad chilled or at room temperature.
- This recipe is packed with nutrients that have been claimed to have fertility-boosting properties, including quinoa (which is high in protein and iron), cherry tomatoes (which are high in lycopene), cucumbers (which are high in antioxidants), red bell peppers (which

are high in vitamin C), and red onions (which are high in folic acid). You can feel free to customize the recipe by adding or subtracting ingredients to suit your taste.

(2)

Ingredients:
- 1 cup cooked black beans
- 1 cup cooked brown rice
- 1/2 cup diced avocado
- 1/2 cup diced mango
- 1/2 cup diced red bell pepper
- 1/4 cup chopped fresh cilantro
- 2 tablespoons olive oil
- 1 tablespoon lime juice
- Salt and pepper to taste

Directions:
- In a large bowl, combine the cooked black beans, cooked brown rice, avocado, mango, red bell pepper, and cilantro.
- In a small bowl, whisk together the olive oil, lime juice, salt, and pepper.
- Pour the dressing over the salad and toss to coat.
- Serve the salad chilled or at room temperature.
- This recipe is high in a number of nutrients that have been claimed to have fertility-boosting properties, including black beans (which are high in protein, iron, and folic acid), brown rice (which is high in B vitamins), avocado (which is high in healthy fats and vitamin E), and mango (which is high in vitamin C). As with the previous recipe, you can feel free to customize the recipe by adding or subtracting ingredients to suit your taste

DINNER

(1)

Ingredients:
1 cup quinoa

1 cup water
1 cup broccoli florets
1 cup diced bell peppers
1 cup sliced mushrooms
1 cup diced onions
1 cup diced zucchini
1 cup diced carrots
1 tablespoon olive oil

- 1 teaspoon garlic, minced
- Salt and pepper, to taste
- Optional: 1/2 cup diced tofu or chicken

Instructions:

- Rinse the quinoa in a fine mesh strainer.
- In a medium saucepan, bring the quinoa and water to a boil.
- Reduce the heat to low, cover, and simmer for about 15 minutes, or until the water is absorbed and the quinoa is tender.
- Heat the oil in a large frying pan or wok over medium-high heat.
- Add the garlic and onions and sauté until the onions are translucent.
- Add the broccoli, bell peppers, mushrooms, zucchini, and carrots to the pan and stir-fry until the vegetables are tender.
- Add the cooked quinoa to the pan and stir to combine.
- Season with salt and pepper to taste.
- If using tofu or chicken, add it to the pan and stir-fry until it is cooked through.
- Serve the stir-fry hot.

This stir-fry is a great source of plant-based protein, fiber, and a variety of vitamins and minerals. The quinoa, vegetables, and tofu or chicken are all rich in nutrients that may help support fertility. Enjoy!

(2)

Ingredients:

- 1 cup jasmine rice
- 1 3/4 cups water
- 1 cup diced tofu
- 1 cup sliced bell peppers

- 1 cup sliced carrots
- 1 cup sliced onions
- 1 cup diced tomatoes
- 1 cup sliced bok choy
- 1 tablespoon sesame oil
- 1 tablespoon soy sauce
- 1 teaspoon grated ginger
- Salt and pepper, to taste

Instructions:

- Rinse the rice in a fine mesh strainer.
- In a medium saucepan, bring the rice and water to a boil.
- Reduce the heat to low, cover, and simmer for about 20 minutes, or until the water is absorbed and the rice is tender.
- Heat the sesame oil in a large frying pan or wok over medium-high heat.
- Add the tofu and stir-fry until it is browned on all sides.
- Add the bell peppers, carrots, onions, and ginger to the pan and stir-fry until the vegetables are tender.
- Add the bok choy and tomatoes to the pan and stir-fry until they are wilted.
- Stir in the cooked rice and soy sauce.
- Season with salt and pepper to taste.
- Serve the stir-fry hot.
-

This stir-fry is a great source of plant-based protein, fiber, and a variety of vitamins and minerals. The tofu, vegetables, and rice are all rich in nutrients that may help support fertility. Enjoy!

(3)

Ingredients:

- 1 cup brown rice
- 2 cups water
- 1 cup diced chicken
- 1 cup sliced bell peppers
- 1 cup sliced asparagus
- 1 cup sliced onions

- 1 cup diced pineapple
- 1 tablespoon coconut oil
- 1 tablespoon honey
- 1 teaspoon curry powder
- Salt and pepper, to taste

Instructions:

- Rinse the rice in a fine mesh strainer.
- In a medium saucepan, bring the rice and water to a boil.
- Reduce the heat to low, cover, and simmer for about 45 minutes, or until the water is absorbed and the rice is tender.
- Heat the coconut oil in a large frying pan or wok over medium-high heat.
- Add the chicken and stir-fry until it is cooked through.
- Add the bell peppers, asparagus, and onions to the pan and stir-fry until the vegetables are tender.
- Stir in the pineapple and honey.
- Sprinkle the curry powder over the stir-fry and stir to combine.
- Season with salt and pepper to taste.
- Serve the stir-fry hot.
-

This stir-fry is a great source of protein, fiber, and a variety of vitamins and minerals. The chicken, vegetables, and brown rice are all rich in nutrients that may help support fertility. Enjoy!

(4)

Ingredients:

- 1 cup farro
- 2 cups water
- 1 cup diced shrimp
- 1 cup sliced bell peppers
- 1 cup sliced zucchini
- 1 cup sliced onions
- 1 cup diced tomatoes
- 1 tablespoon avocado oil
- 1 tablespoon lemon juice
- 1 teaspoon dried basil

- Salt and pepper, to taste

Instructions:

1. Rinse the farro in a fine mesh strainer.
2. In a medium saucepan, bring the farro and water to a boil.
3. Reduce the heat to low, cover, and simmer for about 20 minutes, or until the water is absorbed and the farro is tender.
4. Heat the avocado oil in a large frying pan or wok over medium-high heat.
5. Add the shrimp and stir-fry until it is pink and cooked through.
6. Add the bell peppers, zucchini, and onions to the pan and stir-fry until the vegetables are tender.
7. Stir in the tomatoes and lemon juice.
8. Sprinkle the basil over the stir-fry and stir to combine.
9. Season with salt and pepper to taste.
10. Serve the stir-fry hot.

This stir-fry is a great source of protein, fiber, and a variety of vitamins and minerals. The shrimp, vegetables, and farro are all rich in nutrients that may help support fertility. Enjoy!

B. Fertility-Boosting Pasta Dish

Ingredients:

- 1 pound whole grain pasta
- 1 tablespoon olive oil
- 1 small onion, finely chopped
- 2 cloves garlic, minced
- 1 cup cherry tomatoes, halved
- 1 cup cooked black beans
- 1 cup cooked corn
- 1/2 cup chopped fresh basil
- Salt and pepper, to taste

Instructions:

1. Cook the pasta according to the package instructions. Drain and set aside.
2. In a large saucepan, heat the olive oil over medium heat.
3. Add the onion and cook until it becomes translucent, about 5 minutes.

4. Add the garlic and cook for an additional minute.
5. Add the cherry tomatoes, black beans, corn, and basil to the saucepan and cook until the tomatoes are tender, about 5 minutes.
6. Add the cooked pasta to the saucepan and toss everything together. Season with salt and pepper to taste.
7. Serve hot and enjoy!

This pasta dish is a good source of whole grains, which are important for fertility because they provide essential nutrients such as B vitamins and zinc. The black beans and corn are also rich in antioxidants, which can help to improve fertility by reducing oxidative stress in the body. The cherry tomatoes and basil add flavor and nutrition to the dish, making it a tasty and healthy meal option for those trying to boost their fertility.

Snacks

1. **Fertility-Boosting Energy Bites**

(1)

Ingredients:

- 1 cup rolled oats
- 1/2 cup unsalted nut butter (such as almond or peanut butter)
- 1/3 cup honey
- 1/2 cup ground flaxseeds
- 1/2 cup chopped nuts (such as almonds or walnuts)
- 1/2 cup dried fruit (such as apricots or raisins)
- 1 tsp cinnamon

Instructions:

1. In a large mixing bowl, combine the rolled oats, nut butter, honey, ground flaxseeds, chopped nuts, dried fruit, and cinnamon. Mix until well combined.
2. Roll the mixture into bite-sized balls and place them on a parchment-lined baking sheet.
3. Chill the energy bites in the refrigerator for at least 1 hour before serving.
4. Store the energy bites in an airtight container in the refrigerator for up to 1 week.

These energy bites are packed with nutrients that can help boost fertility, such as omega-3 fatty acids (found in flaxseeds and nuts), iron (found in dried fruit), and antioxidants (found in cinnamon). Enjoy them as a healthy snack or pre-workout boost.

(2)

Ingredients

- 1/2 cup raw pepitas
- 1/2 cup raw sunflower seeds
- 1/2 cup raw pistachios
- 1 T maca powder
- 1 T chia seeds
- 10 medjool dates (pits removed)
- 1/2 teaspoon sea salt.
- 2-3 T water

Instructions

1. In a food processor , grind up the pistachios, chia seeds, sunflower seeds, pepitas, sea salt and maca powder to a coarse consistency.
2. Then add in the dates and continue to pulse.
3. Lastly, add in the water, 1 tablespoon at a time until a dough starts to form.
4. Roll into balls and place in the fridge to firm up. It should only take a minute or two.

FERTILITY-BOOSTING TRAIL MIX

(1)

Ingredients:
1 cup raw almonds
1 cup raw pumpkin seeds
1 cup raw sunflower seeds
1 cup dried cranberries
1 cup dark chocolate chips
Instructions:

- Preheat your oven to 300°F (150°C).
- Spread the almonds, pumpkin seeds, and sunflower seeds on a baking sheet and roast for 10-15 minutes or until fragrant.
- Allow the nuts and seeds to cool completely.
- In a large mixing bowl, combine the cooled nuts and seeds with the dried cranberries and dark chocolate chips.
- Store the trail mix in an airtight container at room temperature for up to 1 month.

This trail mix is a healthy snack that is packed with nutrients that can support fertility. For example, almonds are a good source of
zinc, which is important for reproductive health, and pumpkin seeds are high in omega-3 fatty acids, which are important for hormone production. Sunflower seeds are a good source of vitamin E, which is important for maintaining a healthy reproductive system, and cranberries are high in antioxidants, which can help to reduce oxidative stress on the body. Dark chocolate is also high in antioxidants and has been shown to have a number of health benefits, including improving blood flow to the reproductive organs

(2)

Ingredients:
- 1 cup raw nuts (almonds, Brazil nuts, macadamia nuts, etc.)
- 1/2 cup seeds (pumpkin seeds, sunflower seeds, etc.)
- 1/2 cup dried fruit (raisins, cranberries, goji berries, etc.)
- 1/4 cup cocoa nibs or chocolate chips (optional)

Instructions:
1. Mix all ingredients together in a large bowl.
2. Transfer the mixture to an airtight container or a resealable bag.
3. Enjoy as a snack or sprinkle over oatmeal, yogurt, or smoothies.

This trail mix is high in nutrients that are important for fertility, such as healthy fats, protein, and antioxidants. The nuts and seeds provide
healthy fats and protein, which are important for hormone production and healthy ovulation. The dried fruit is a good source of antioxidants, which can help to reduce inflammation and improve fertility. The cocoa nibs or

chocolate chips (if using) add a touch of sweetness and can also be a good source of antioxidants. Enjoy!

CHAPTER THREE

FERTILITY-BOOSTING HERBS AND SPICES

There are several herbs and spices that have been traditionally used to boost fertility and improve reproductive health. Here are a few examples:

Maca root : This herb is native to the Andes and has been used for centuries to improve fertility and increase libido. It is believed to help regulate hormones and improve ovarian function.

Fenugreek : This spice has been shown to improve reproductive health in men and women. It is believed to increase testosterone levels in men and improve ovarian function in women.

Red clover : This herb is rich in phytoestrogens, which are plant-based compounds that mimic the effects of estrogen in the body. It is believed to help regulate hormones and improve fertility.

Ashwagandha : This herb is an adaptogen, which means it helps the body adapt to stress. It is believed to improve fertility by reducing stress and improving reproductive health.

Ginger : This spice has anti-inflammatory properties and is believed to improve blood flow to the reproductive organs, which may improve fertility.

It is important to note that the effectiveness of these herbs and spices in boosting fertility has not been extensively studied and more research is needed. It is always a good idea to speak with a healthcare provider before starting any new supplement or herbal regimen..

6 KITCHEN HERBS AND SPICES TO BOOST FERTILITY

We tend to suppose medicinal sauces as being fully different than culinary sauces, but that's not always the case.

The great thing about kitchen sauces is you do n't need to study clinical herbalism to take full advantage of their health and fertility benefits. Just open your closet and fridge, add some flavor to your food, belt some succulent teas, and savor every bite & drop.

Then there are many kitchen sauces to consider if fertility health is on your mind.

1. Garlic

Garlic is the ubiquitous condiment used by nearly every culture. all over the world, folks turn to it to add some serious flavor to food. Plus it's one of the most extensively used medicinal sauces.

It relaxes your blood vessels and promotes rotation, and good blood inflow is vital to keeping your organs in tip top shape, including your ovaries and uterus. For the guys, acceptable blood inflow is necessary for constructions.

How to use

- Add diced cloves to stir- feasts, mists, and pesto.
- Rub a cut clove over chuck or indeed in a coliseum just before adding haze or salad to it.
- Inoculate olive oil painting with many cloves to use anytime a form or mess calls for a mizzle of EVOO.

2. gusto

gusto is without question a succulent condiment that can be fluently added to a number of refections and drinks, and helps alleviate period cramps and nausea during gestation. It's high in antioxidants, which plays a defensive part for your ovaries and eggs from oxidative damage and stress. numerous herbalists also say it increases blood inflow to your lady corridor, delivering important nutrients and clearing down poisons.

How to use

- Tear about a thumb size quantum and add it to hot cereals.
- Add a1/2 inch hulled piece to a smoothie.
- Make into a delicious tea. Add bomb and honey or just enjoy as is.

3. Turmeric

Turmeric, the golden child of Ayurveda, protects your DNA from damage, acts as an anti-inflammatory, and protects your liver. With your liver playing a veritably important part in detoxification and hormonal health, keeping it healthy and happy is pivotal to both fertility and your overall heartiness.

How to use

- Add1/8-1/ 4 tsp to smoothies.
- Combine with your favorite sweet spices, especially pepper, and add to sauteed vegetables.
- Stir a bit into rice or quinoa for flavor and color that just wo n't quit.

4. Cayenne

Cayenne has a character among herbalist as adding just as important heat to your libido as it does to your food. It's regarded as an aphrodisiac, able to add sexual desire and flavoring up your coitus life.

Whether or not any of that's true, is debatable, but what we do know is that cayenne has been shown to appreciatively impact energy metabolism. The strong association between energy metabolism, hormonal regulation, and womanish reduplication makes cayenne a helpful kitchen spice for fertility.

How to use

- Sprinkle(and I do mean sprinkle, this stuff is potent) on avocado toast.
- Add a gusto to hot chocolate.
- Stir a bit into peanut adulation with a little cinnamon for a new spin on an old favorite- apple and peanut adulation. Or try this seasoned peanut adulation blend on a baked sweet potato. tasteful!

5. Cinnamon

Who does n't love the sweet smell of cinnamon? Despite advancing a subtle agreeableness to foods and drinks, cinnamon can actually help homogenize blood sugar. Balanced blood sugar can help ameliorate overall hormonal balance, especially for those with fertility issues due to PCOS.

How to use

- Sprinkle on hot cereals.

- Add to apple(or pear) and peanut adulation.

6. Nettles

Nettles really do n't get enough attention. They 're protean, easy to use, and chock full of health benefits. It's full of factory- grounded,non-heme iron, one of the micronutrients that have been linked to drop the chance of ovulatory infertility .

How to use

- Make a simple tea or infusion to belt throughout the day.
- Add to smoothies, mists, and stews.
- Brume and eat as a succulent side dish.
- Have delightful exploring your closet and fridge. Just a sprinkle and a pinch will do to add fun and variety to your reflections.

CHAPTER FOUR

FERTILITY-BOOSTING LIFESTYLE TIPS

KEYS TO FERTILITY

For both women and men, the keys to fertility include maintaining a healthy weight, exercising, and choosing foods that support your capability to conceive and achieve gestation.

30% of infertility has been associated with weight axes. infertility rates are 3 times advanced in fat women. Women who are fat can ameliorate their fertility by losing just 5 of their body weight. Insulin resistance causes the body to release further insulin which halts ovulation. Light women frequently suffer from ovulation problems as well.

Obesity in men alters testosterone and other hormones that can affect sperm count and sperm mobility. Sperm- related infertility accounts for over to 33 of manly factor infertility .

In addition to diet, life choices that support generalizations include limiting alcohol consumption, quitting smoking, and moderate diurnal exercise.

Healthy Eating Can Optimize Fertility

What you eat affects the health of you or your mate's eggs and sperm. A Harvard study reported that women can drop infertility due to ovulation diseases by 80% with healthy salutary changes

NINE(9) SPECIFIC RECOMMENDATIONS

Consuming full- fat dairy is associated with a lower threat of ovarian dysfunction and supports healthy ovulation. Avoid Low- fat dairy because studies have shown they increase ovulatory dysfunction.

- Consume protein from meat and vegetables. Do n't eat too important beast protein as it increases the threat of infertility .
- Consuming soy can help womanish fertility. Men should avoid soy as it can lower sperm count.
- Eat further fiber.
- Eat dark leafy flora to ameliorate ovulation, and make healthy sperm.
- Include sap in your diet as they boost fertility.
- Adding walnuts to your man's diet can ameliorate his fertility.
- Avoid Trans Fats which are associated with a high threat of infertility .
- Avoid Largely reused foods and hydrogenated canvases .
- Reduce carbs and sugar. Eat complex carbs to stabilize blood sugar situations. High blood sugar situations have been reported to reduce generality.
- Moderate caffeine consumption of 1- 2 mugs per day has no effect on fertility. Advanced boluses may. The wisdom isn't conclusive.
  1. **Antenatal Vitamins**

- Take a multivitamin or antenatal vitamin that's formulated to give the nutrients you need for optimal hormone function, egg development, and fetal development. Antenatal vitamins contain folate, Vitamins A&D, iron, B6, and B12. These nutrients are the structure blocks of a healthy gestation. Folate from food alone isn't sufficient. Folate from nutritive supplements can increase gestation success. Women should take 800 mcg/ day of folate during fertility treatments and throughout gestation.

- Take an iron supplement. Studies report that women who regularly took an iron supplement were 40 less likely to have difficulty getting pregnant.
- Sperm stored in the body is at threat of oxidative stress which damages sperm DNA. The threat for damage to sperm involves smoking, obesity , habitual complaint, and being over the age of 38. Including antioxidants like vitamin C, E, Folic Acid, selenium, and zinc can reduce sperm damage.
- Vitamin D is essential to the creation of coitus hormones, and for ovulation. Lower vitamin D affects sperm motility, and in women is associated with gestation complications. A Yale study reported that vitamin D insufficiency is linked to infertility . perfecting Vitamin D situations has been shown to ameliorate success with IVF.
- Vitamin E is associated with positive reproductive issues. It can dock the time to gestation, and ameliorate sperm motility. But take caution since high boluses of these supplements can have a negative impact. Omega 3 adipose acids help regulate your hormones, promote ovulation and ameliorate blood inflow to the reproductive organs.

2. **Exercise**

Moderate exercise (up to one hour) can reduce the risk of pregnancy complications and improve sperm quality, which can lead to successful pregnancies. However, exercising for less than 15 minutes can increase the risk of pregnancy complications, and extreme exercise can also cause pregnancy issues. The way you exercise can also impact your success with in vitro fertilization (IVF).

3. **Oral health**

Good oral health is important because conditions such as gum disease, depression, and periodontitis can negatively affect pregnancy.

4. **Quit smoking**

Studies show that smoking increases the risk of pregnancy by 13% and can prolong the time it takes to conceive. It also increases the risk of delivery complications and can cause birth defects.

5. **Alcohol**

Alcohol can affect both male and female fertility, impacting fertility and implantation. There is no safe level of alcohol consumption when trying to conceive.

6. **Stress**

Stress can impair fertility, but techniques such as acupuncture, yoga, meditation, breathing exercises, and other mind-body therapies can help. Massage can also be beneficial.

7. **Timing intercourse**

Understanding your fertility cycle can increase your chances of conceiving, and timing intercourse can help improve the chances of pregnancy, but it does not affect fertility.

8. **Lubricant**

It is known that certain water-based lubricants and lubricants that contain a spermicide should be avoided, but there are sperm-friendly lubricants that will not affect sperm motility. Melatonin is produced naturally by the body during sleep, but artificial light, including the light from device screens, can affect its production.

9. **Sleep**

Getting enough sleep can also reduce cortisol levels, which can increase testosterone.

Men can improve their fertility by avoiding tight-fitting clothing, long bike rides, and hot tubs, and by not placing laptops on their lap, as this can increase scrotal temperature and decrease sperm production.